My Son: Living Life With Down Syndrome

My Son: Living Life With Down Syndrome

First Year of Life

Amy Sprague

iUniverse, Inc.
New York Lincoln Shanghai

My Son: Living Life With Down Syndrome

First Year of Life

iUniverse books may be ordered through booksellers or by contacting:

iUniverse
2021 Pine Lake Road, Suite 100
Lincoln, NE 68512
www.iuniverse.com
1-800-Authors (1-800-288-4677)

ISBN-13: 978-0-595-37403-8 (pbk)
ISBN-13: 978-0-595-81797-9 (ebk)
ISBN-10: 0-595-37403-4 (pbk)
ISBN-10: 0-595-81797-1 (ebk)

Printed in the United States of America

At 23 years old, I never expected my life to change so dramatically in a year's time. For me, what was supposed to be a new and exciting change in so little time became a struggle with much fear, emptiness, and sadness within.

On November 30th, 2003, I found out that I was going to be a mother. Tears of joy ran down my face with feelings of happiness that overwhelmed me. Here I am a soon-to-be mother with a child growing inside.

Throughout my pregnancy I had doubts going through my mind. Would I be able to take care of my newborn? Would I be financially stable enough to take care of him/her? Would I be able to provide for all of its needs?

Those thoughts went through my mind several times. At one point I even thought about giving my child up for adoption because I wanted him/her to have so much and didn't think I would be able to take care of a child on my own, either mentally and physically.

As months passed, I began to feel feelings inside me that I never thought could be possible. I could feel my child moving around and kicking. Those feelings were so amazing and to think how something so small and remarkable could be able to do all this in such a tiny space amazed me.

I began to get further and further along in my pregnancy. I started picking out boy and girl names, but for some reason I had a strong instinct that I was going to have a boy. I picked four names that I liked, but the name that stuck in my head was the name Cooper. It was a name that you didn't hear very often and it sounded unique. Now it was time to try to figure out some middle names. Right off, the middle name Allen came to mind and it just stuck, so now I had my boy name picked out. It would be Cooper Allen Sprague. Before I knew it, the time arrived for me to find out the sex of my child. I was so excited and still kept telling myself I was going to have a boy. When the doctors confirmed from the ultrasound that it was a boy, I was so happy and excited, I couldn't wait to tell everyone what I was having and the name that I had chosen.

At that point I decided I was going to keep my child. All I could do was to try to do the best that I could on my own. I got to the point where I couldn't see turning my back on my son when I'd come this far. I knew that there was going to be a lot of work involved and that my life would change so much by having a child. But I knew I could do it even if it meant my going without to make sure my son was well off.

Little did I know that what the future had in store for me was more than anyone could ever imagine. By the time I was about eight months along, the doctor performed a test called an AFP (alpha fetal protein) test. The test was a blood test that would be taken from me to determine if my unborn child would have any abnormalities such as Down Syndrome or spinal bifida, etc. The results of the test would take approximately two weeks to come back because of its being sent out of state.

When two weeks passed, I called my OB doctor to see if the results of my lab test were back. While waiting on hold I kept saying to myself, everything please be fine, please don't let my child have anything wrong. When the nurse came back on she informed me that my lab test came back normal and they found nothing wrong with my child. At that point, I let out a big sigh of relief and now could look forward to delivering a healthy baby boy.

It was now time to get things together that I needed for when it was time to deliver my son. I already had Cooper's changing table and crib, but needed to buy some clothes, diapers, a bath tub and accessories, etc. I was so excited to be able to go clothes shopping; just seeing all the cute clothes they had brought tears to my eyes. I could even picture my baby wearing them.

I gave some money to my friend Kelley because she had to go to Presque Isle anyway, so she picked out some clothes, bought Cooper's bath tub, bath supplies, baby wipes, and diapers for me. Heck, she even went out of her way and spent her money and got Cooper a few clothes.

When the time for my final checkup arrived, my doctor set me up for some Non-Stress Tests. At this point, all the tests were coming out normal and fine until Thursday, August 12, 2004, at 1:30 p.m.

About an hour prior to my test I had a checkup with the doctor and everything seemed okay. Just when I thought I could go home after having my Non-Stress Test, the doctors wanted to keep an eye on me for a little while longer before they let me go home. What happened was that right at the end of the test they noticed that Cooper's heart rate had dropped.

After an hour of observation I asked if I would be able to go home. When my doctor came into the room, she informed me that she would like to keep me for the weekend and that if I hadn't delivered by Monday, they were going to induce labor. The thought went through my head, Is my child okay? Is there possibly something wrong and they don't want to tell me? I tried to stay calm but all I could think about was whether everything would be okay.

When my doctor came back into the room to see how I was doing and check the contractions and heart rate monitor, she told me that she felt that I would not be having my child that night. So they then moved me into another room.

By 7:00 p.m. I began to slowly feel more and more contractions and pressure. It wasn't anything major at that time, but I had a feeling that the doctor was wrong and that I was going to have my child that night.

Come 12:00 midnight, there were no ifs, ands or buts; my son wanted out and he wanted it to be soon. I called up my friend Kelley and spoke with her. She had a feeling all along that I was going to have him on Friday the 13th, the one day I didn't want to have him on. However, she told me that she would be up around 1 p.m. When she arrived, she also had her sister and nephew with her.

Before I knew it, the contractions began to get more and more intense and soon it was time to start pushing. Then at 3:41 a.m. on Friday, August 13th, 2004, I welcomed into the world my son Cooper Allen Sprague.

At first, I didn't hear a cry from him but that was because they were suctioning him out. Cooper had inhaled some meconium. Then when I heard his first cry, I cried. When the nurse brought Cooper over for me to hold, I welcomed my little angel into the world. I was so exhausted and tired that I held him for only a few seconds, and then they took Cooper off to the nursery.

Cooper entered the world weighing in at seven pounds three ounces and he measured eighteen-and-a-half inches long. Once born, Cooper developed mild respiratory distress, requiring oxygen and an evaluation.

When the nurse came back in we delivered the placenta and she stitched me up. Then off to my room I went. I said goodnight to my friends and thanked them for coming. They stayed about a half hour longer to see Cooper, and then they too went home.

The next day arrived quickly. I went into the nursery to see how Cooper was doing. He was weaned off oxygen and antibiotics. Cooper was the only baby that was born that night and that was also in the nursery. The pediatrician on call looked over Cooper and talked with me about Cooper's platelet count. She told me that Cooper's count was really low and that it continued to drop.

As the following days passed, Cooper's platelet count continued to drop even more. His pediatrician and I were becoming very worried. Cooper's count got to the point where it was only 30,000, when the count is supposed to be between 130,000 and 400,000.

By Monday, August 16th, Cooper's platelet count still wasn't improving. Cooper's doctor informed me that she felt that Cooper should go to Eastern Maine Medical Center in Bangor to have more thorough tests done. She also informed me that she felt Cooper potentially may have had the need for a platelet transfusion.

I was so scared when she told me the news. The thought of a baby going through a transfusion made me even more upset. I paced the floor and called a friend for support. I never once imagined that in such a short little time here on earth a newborn would have to go through so much.

When the ambulance came I could feel my heart racing; seeing Cooper in an incubator hurt me. I felt so hopeless and unable to help him. Here was my son, unaware of what's going on and extremely hungry, and he couldn't eat yet because the doctors were worried the long ride could make him sick.

As we pulled out of the hospital's entrance, thoughts went through my mind of what would happen if he did need a transfusion. And what if he caught something from the blood? Many scary thoughts ran through my mind but they weren't as bad as the EMTs turning on their sirens and flashing lights off and on all the way there. I kept thinking to myself, with the sounds of the sirens going off, what if my child doesn't make it to the hospital?

Two hours later, when we finally arrived at Eastern Maine Medical Center, I had the doctors check Cooper in and get him situated. I then went and checked into the local Ronald McDonald House only a couple minutes away from the hospital.

An hour later I returned to the hospital where I met at the NICU (Neonatal Intensive Care Unit) two genetic counselors. They sat down with me and explained to me briefly about a chromosome test they were performing on Cooper for trisomy 21.

They said it was because Cooper was showing some signs of having Down Syndrome. The test results would let me know tomorrow. Cooper's features included a transverse palmar crease, or simian crease (a small crease across the center of the palms of the hands), a wide space between his big toe and second toe, and small ears that sat low.

I kept telling myself that everything would be okay and that Cooper was going to be fine. The next morning I met again with the team.

They informed me of some good news: Cooper's platelet count had spontaneously gone back up. But the news that was about to hit me was more than I could handle and it changed my life forever.

At that point, Cooper was having an echocardiogram done on his heart by the cardiologist; while that was taking place the team informed me that Cooper did indeed have trisomy 21 and he also had two holes in his heart that would later on need surgery.

The genetics team informed me that they felt Cooper's trisomy 21 result was a fluke because when they tested his chromosomes, Cooper did not carry the gene called translocation trisomy 21, which means that if indeed he had this gene it would have been inherited through the father or me.

Then he explained to me Cooper's heart conditions and he drew me a little diagram so I could better understand what was going on.

When and if Cooper would need surgery, they would have to patch the ASD (atrial septal defect) and the VSD (ventricular septal defect).

When there is a large defect between the atria, a large amount of oxygen-rich (red) blood from the heart's left side leaks back to the right side. Then it is pumped back to the lungs even though it's already been refreshed with oxygen. This is inefficient, since the blood that's already been to the lungs is returning there, and blood that needs to go to the lungs is being displaced. This is what was happening with Cooper's ASD.

When there's a large opening between the ventricles, a large amount of oxygen-rich (red) blood from the heart's left side is forced through the defect to the right side. Then it's pumped back to the lungs, even though it's already been refreshed with oxygen. This is inefficient, since blood that needs to go to the lungs is being displaced. The heart, which has to pump an extra amount of blood, is over-worked and may enlarge. This is what was happening with Cooper's VSD.

Hearing all of this news all together in the time span of about ten minutes was so overwhelming, I didn't even know what to say or think. I felt so scared, hopeless, and alone. But mostly I was worried about what was going on with my son.

I never even knew or heard of Down Syndrome until then; I didn't even know what a child with this condition would grow up to look like or become.

Thoughts were going through my head: Will Cooper live to have a normal and happy life? Will he be able to graduate from high school, play sports or even get through school without being teased and made fun of?

It was all too much for me to absorb, so I decided to go back to the Ronald McDonald House for the night, and I informed Cooper's doctors that I would be back in the morning. I needed time to think things over and make sure that I wasn't upset, because I knew Cooper could sense it if I were.

All night long I felt so lonely and empty inside. With much hurt and regret, I kept blaming myself and asking, What did I do to deserve this? Why me?

For that whole night I cried till I cried myself asleep. When I awakened the next morning, I cried once again, then asked myself over and over, How will I be able to take care of him? Will I be able to provide him with all of the special care he will need?

Upon entering Cooper's room I met the genetics team. The worker had given me a book called *Babies with Down Syndrome, A New Parents' Guide*.

To me, the book was way too confusing to understand or even to read. It had so many medical terms, but never once did it explain a parent's point of view of what to expect or how as a parent they dealt with all the changes.

Then the teams had also talked to me about many organizations out there for adoption that take children with special needs and find a loving and caring home for them when a parent can't or doesn't want to provide for the child.

I sat back and once again thoughts were going through my head: Maybe it would be a good idea to give Cooper up; this way he would get all the help and medical attention he needs.

After the team left, I held and fed my son. When I looked at him tears formed; I didn't know what I should do. Here I am a single mother with a sick child; what am I to do?

While holding Cooper, I thought to myself, How can I turn my back on him, especially knowing how special he is?

I just couldn't give him up. I was heartbroken, still feeling much guilt and hatred, thinking that it was my fault and that I was to blame for Cooper having Down Syndrome.

I lay Cooper back in his bed as I waited for a nurse to walk by so I could find out when we would be able to go home.

Once I met up with the nurse she told me that if Cooper continued to do well, then not tomorrow, but the next day he would be able to go home.

Hearing that made me realize that soon I'd be bringing him home and soon the journey would begin for both of us. I decided that I would go back to the Ronald McDonald House for the night and make some phone calls so that everything would be set when we got home.

The first thing I did was call my friend Kelley and told her the good news. She and her sister Sandy went over to my apartment and set up the crib and changing table for my son so it would be all done when he came home.

I also had discussed with Kelley about her possibly being able to drive to Bangor to pick up Cooper and me upon discharge and explained that I needed his car seat so he could be fitted in it.

Kelley had agreed to pick us up. I told her that I would get back to her the next day regarding when we would be able to leave.

Next I called my parents in Vermont to tell them the good news about us going home. My parents and I discussed their driving up to see Cooper. We then made plans for the following week to visit.

Once all my phone calls were done I was pretty much exhausted and ready for bed. This time my head was clearer and I knew I'd be able to sleep with no problems.

The next morning when I got up I thanked the staff for all their help and support. I had never heard of their program until it came down to the point where I actually had to use them.

I am so thankful that there is such a program out there for families to turn to. If it weren't for all their help and support, I don't know what I would have done or who I would have been able to turn to.

The sad part of the whole thing is that the Ronald McDonald House makes its earnings only by donations and collecting pull tabs from cans, and even that isn't much. I wished that there was some way I would be able to help them. One of these days I know I'll be able to donate some money in thanks.

The Ronald McDonald House helps so many people in tragic situations, ranging from children being in the hospital to people going through chemotherapy.

After my talk with the staff, I signed out, wished everyone the best of luck, and headed back to the hospital, where I would be spending the night with my son taking full care of him before we went home.

I walked into Cooper's room with so much happiness inside that the day was almost here for us to go home.

It had been a long week and I had found out and learned so much in that short time about my son. Even though I had no idea what the future would hold for us, all I knew was that I would love and take care of my son no matter what.

It took me a while to realize how much I was going to change. I had to grow up in so many ways. Now it wasn't just me to look out for—I had an innocent little baby now to take care of. The responsibilities would be an endless job but I was more than willing and ready to step up to the plate.

That night, taking care of Cooper by myself for the first time made me grow even closer to him. I felt an instant special bond between us that words can't even describe. The night went really well even though Cooper, like most babies, slept through most of the night. His feedings were okay. Cooper would drink about 2–3 oz. of his formula while falling asleep halfway through it.

It was weird, though, because I had expected to hear the cries of a baby throughout the night, yet I lucked out because Cooper would rarely cry. I knew that soon we would be home and then our journey could begin, where we both would learn things from one another.

The next day didn't come fast enough for me I was so excited and impatient to take Cooper home. That morning when I woke up, I fed and changed Cooper and brought him back into the NICU until the time came for us to go home.

Today was the day that not only would I be bringing my son home, but I would also be giving Cooper his first bath. I was so excited but scared to death—I was afraid of hurting him. The nurses stood by and helped show me different ways I could bathe him as well as how to clean his umbilical cord.

When the nurse had mentioned to me that within a week or so his cord would fall off on its own, the first thing that went through my mind was, Would it be painful? And yuck. The nurse informed me that Cooper would not feel any pain and it would be okay.

I finally got word that at 11:00 a.m. Cooper would have his car seat safety test, which would last an hour, then we would be able to go home as long as everything continued to go smoothly.

I stepped out of the room to call Kelley and inform her that we would be discharged at approximately 12:00 noon, but I would need Cooper's car seat by 11:00 a.m.

Watching the clock and counting down the hours, then minutes, took forever, but I became more and more excited for the journey home.

While I was waiting for my friend to show up with Cooper's car seat, I watched a few movies. One was the car seat safety video; then I watched movies about how to take care of your newborn and bathing videos.

Cooper was sound asleep and looked so peaceful and content. I couldn't wait to pull back into my home's driveway. Before I knew it, the time arrived for his car seat test. When I saw my friend Kelley I was so happy and excited; it seemed like forever since I had seen her or talked to her.

Kelley went over and saw little Cooper and showed me the clothes she'd picked out for him to come home in. The clothes were so adorable; it was Cooper's Winnie The Pooh set. While the nurses bundled Cooper in his car seat to begin the hour-long test, we went out to lunch in town.

When we arrived back to the hospital it was almost time to take Cooper home. When I put on his little hat it was so funny because there wasn't one that could fit onto his tiny little head. Before I knew it, it was time to finally go home. While Kelley went to get her car, I signed Cooper's release papers.

Just as we were getting ready to exit the hospital a doctor stopped us in the hallway, which was a very good thing. The doctor had forgotten to take off Cooper's security band and if it had gone off, all the sirens and alarms would have gone off throughout the hospital and the doors would have shut and locked, and then the police would have been on the scene in a heartbeat. I never laughed so hard in my life but was very thankful he stopped us in time, because I know I would have had a heart attack if something like that were to have happened, and can you imagine how Cooper would have reacted?

When we walked out of the hospital together, I let out a big sigh of relief as I walked Cooper to the car and buckled him in. I was so proud and happy that this moment had finally arrived.

Two and a half hours later, when I finally arrived back on familiar ground, that's when the happiness really took over. I was tired from the long trip and couldn't wait to see how my place looked, especially Cooper's room.

When I walked through my apartment doors, I was welcomed home by my next-door neighbors and my downstairs neighbor. All I could say was it felt so good to be home. I knew I was going to look things over in my place, get my son out of his car seat and into his crib, then I was going to lie down and take a nap while I could.

So far, the first day at home went really well. I noticed Cooper spent a lot of time sleeping, but I knew that he would be anyway, being a newborn. In a way, it seemed good because this way I got the chance to catch up on some much-needed and well-deserved sleep as well.

As the days went by, Cooper's feedings started to become hard for him. He would drink only half an ounce of formula every three hours, and was constantly sleeping. It would even get to the point where he would fall asleep in the middle of eating and/or not even wake up to be fed. I knew something was wrong but didn't know what. I figured I would wait until after my parents visited, and if Cooper continued to do poorly with his feedings, I would get him in to see his doctor as soon as possible.

When my family came up from Vermont, they were so excited and happy to meet and welcome their grandson into the world. He was so small and fragile, but so peaceful and quiet. You hardly even heard a cry out of him.

Still eating poorly, I decided it was time to take Cooper in to the doctors. Once in the doctor's office, his doctor looked him over and weighed him. At this point, Cooper was starting to lose weight. I informed her that Cooper wouldn't eat much, that he would fall asleep during his feedings, and would not wake up in the middle of the night to be fed.

I also told her how my friends and I tried everything to get his attention and wake him up, like tickling him, shaking bags, or even slapping our hands on the table. Nothing was going to wake up Cooper out of his dead sleep. She then decided to admit him into the hospital to find out what was going on. I felt like I was a bad mother and that everyone thought I wasn't feeding my child.

Come to find out, it was a good thing we admitted Cooper. They got to see firsthand what I was experiencing at home, and that what I was saying was the truth. But the news I was about to be told struck me hard and I didn't know what to do but cry.

The doctor informed me that Cooper was experiencing heart failure, though it didn't seem too bad at that time. That was why he would sleep all the time and give me such a hard time with his feedings. I didn't know what to say or even think at that point; I just wanted Cooper to be alright. I was not expecting that anything like this would ever happen anytime soon. The doctors continued to monitor Cooper and keep a close eye on him.

The next day, on my way back home from visiting Cooper, just as I walked through my door I received a phone call that a parent should never have to hear.

"Amy, you need to come back to the hospital. Cooper is in heart failure and needs to be air-flown down state for surgery. He is blue and on oxygen; he was fine one minute, then turned for the worse."

Tears ran from my face as panic began to set in. I was so scared and afraid I was going to lose my son. I got a ride from my neighbor back up to the hospital. I ran all the way down the hall until I got to the nursery.

When I saw my little angel all hooked up to monitors and on oxygen, I lost it. His doctor told me that now is the time for his surgery and that if he didn't get it right then he would probably die.

I then lost it. I began crying frantically, not knowing what to do or even to whom I should turn. I called my friend Kelley and she came up to see him while we were waiting for Life Flight to come.

Cooper looked so helpless and he was crying. The oxygen tent they had over him was making him very mad. Cooper had his pacifier but kept losing it, which made him even more upset, and then he kept trying to pull the tent off him. I wanted so badly to be able to pick him up and comfort him, but all I could do was talk to him and rub his legs.

When Life Flight arrived, I was panicking because I couldn't go down with him due to there not being enough room. Payday was at least three weeks away and I had no money.

My son was about to go to Portland and the Maine Medical Center. Here I was stranded with no way to be by my child's side, not knowing if he would make it through the weekend or even through the night.

The doctors informed me that they would call me if anything happened and that when they arrived at the hospital they would make sure someone would call and let me know. I left them my phone number and Kelley's. I told them that I would most likely be at her house.

When the EMTs took Cooper away I cried even harder, unsure of how he was and wanting so badly to be by his side. When I got to Kelley's house, all I could think about was Cooper. Is he okay? Will he survive the flight? And will he hang on until I can get there to be by his side? I felt so hopeless and unable to help my son. I didn't even know if I was coming or going.

Finally, two and a half hours later, I received a phone call from the hospital telling me that Cooper made it safely and that they were getting him situated in his room. The nurse told me that I could call any time to see how he was doing and that they would take really good care of him.

I swear that night and the whole weekend I must have called the hospital every one to two hours to check up on Cooper. I think they were even getting tired of my calling because a nurse told me if anything were to happen they had my number and that Cooper was doing okay. But I had to hear it for myself that he was fine.

I wasn't trying to be a pain, but having my son so far away from me and hanging on to life by a thread worried me. I was so afraid that if Cooper passed away I wouldn't be there to spend as much time with him as I could. Just thinking about that was so scary. I tried everything and anything to find a way to buy a bus ticket down. Finally, when I was about to give up, good news came my way and a friend came through with the money for a bus ticket.

When I arrived at the Portland bus terminal, I called a cab to pick me up to go to the hospital. I was new to the area and had no idea how big Portland was. When I arrived at Barbara Bush Children's Hospital at Maine Medical Center, I asked the front desk how to get to the Barbara Bush inpatient unit where Cooper was staying. The name Barbara Bush Children's Hospital was chosen when suggested during a campaign while they were building the hospital.

The hospital was so big it had many winding, long hallways, with several elevators and 7–8 different floors. I felt so lost and I knew that in the hospital if you didn't know your way around and stopped to ask for help, it would be very easy to get lost. I must have stopped and asked directions at least four different times. When I arrived at the wing, I checked in and had to get a parents' pass.

When I got to see my son, I was so happy to be there but sad as well, because Cooper was so sick and had lost a lot more weight, weighing in now at a little more than five pounds. The nurses told me that Cooper was doing fine and how he was such a cute, happy baby and that they hardly heard a peep or cry out of him.

Later that evening, when I got to meet with Cooper's pediatrician cardiologist, he informed me that they would like to see Cooper gain a little weight before they did the surgery, so that way, the chances of him making it through the post-op would be greater.

I was so nervous and upset at the thought that my helpless, sick little boy needed to have a major surgery that could cost him his life. I kept telling myself that he would be fine and that from day one Cooper had been a fighter. I wasn't about to turn and walk away, especially knowing my son needed me the most, more now than ever.

The doctors informed me that they were looking at doing his surgery a week later. I visited with my son for a few hours and then I had to go to the local Ronald McDonald House and check in. Luckily, they let me stay there while Cooper was in the hospital. It was perfect because the hospital was only about three blocks away. So walking there and back would be so much easier, even though at nighttime walking there and back seemed a little scary, especially in a new and big town.

My stay for the first few days at the Ronald McDonald House felt uncomfortable. After time, I got to meet some really cool people and find out other families' situations. One of the families I met had twin girls that were born prematurely with a lot of health problems; I met another family whose daughter was in a horrible car accident and was badly injured.

Over time, I began to grow close relationships with everyone, including the staff members. The staff really made me feel at home and the atmosphere was like a home setting. It was cool, because every Friday night we all got pizza delivered for free to the House for supper, and then about every other night a bunch of volunteers would get together and make a very nice meal for us at suppertime.

It was nice; heck, we even had one morning where some restaurant owners and workers came to the House and made us all a homemade breakfast with toast, pancakes, bacon, sausage, eggs, and bagels. It really felt good to know that there are people out there who care about those families who are in a saddened situation.

We all became such good friends that every time we saw one another we would ask how everyone was doing as well as their children, and at nighttime almost every night we got together when we could to watch the baseball playoffs on T.V. It got really interesting at times because half the room would be White Sox fans and the other half Red Sox. But we all had a blast. It was our time to relax and try to get our minds off things for a little while.

As the weeks progressed, Cooper's eating habits were slowly declining and his weight was staying stable. It was now to the point where it was time to do the surgery or he would end up dying.

When the appointed day came for Cooper's open-heart surgery, he was seven weeks old. My mom and dad came up from Vermont to be by my side and support me through the rough day I was about to have.

On the morning of his surgery, I was so nervous and upset. I didn't want to see Cooper go, but I knew it was all in God's hands now. But I also had to keep telling myself that he's a fighter, he will make it. When I held Cooper in my arms for the last time before they took him to pre-op, I was so scared I didn't even want to let him go. I cried so much, and to walk away from him was very hard for me.

I knew that the waiting game would take a toll on me as I waited to hear updates on my son. I know I was constantly passing the floors and must have smoked at least two packs of cigarettes. When my parents finally arrived around 1:00 p.m., it was an hour after Cooper went into pre-op. Seeing them made me feel a little more at ease and happy because I wouldn't be going through this totally alone.

When they walked through the waiting room I quickly gave them both a hug and kiss as I tried my hardest to hold back tears. Hours passed by as I paced the floor. We all went to the cafeteria to get some lunch. When we arrived back at the waiting room, I still didn't hear anything about Cooper's condition.

Cooper was supposed to be out of surgery and in the ICU (intensive care unit) by 4:00 p.m. That time had come, but there was still no news about my son.

Still passing the floors and at this point getting really worried that something bad had happened to my son, I played some cards with my folks to try to get my mind off things. At that point, I became more and more nervous; my body got to the point where it was shaking because I had no idea if Cooper was even still alive.

By 6:00 p.m. I finally received a phone call from the surgeon's nurse. She informed me that Cooper was doing fine but they had to go back in because the hole that they patched had a small leak and they were not sure where it was coming from.

At this point I almost panicked; Mom and Dad kept me calm. All I could think about was that the patch wasn't going to hold or that Cooper would end up bleeding to death.

Eight p.m. arrived and I still heard no news about Cooper's condition. Then by 8:15 p.m. the phone rang. When I answered, it was the surgeon's nurse once again to inform me that Cooper was doing well and was out of surgery. They were finishing the stitches, would bandage him up, and then once he got up to the ICU in about fifteen minutes, I would be able to see him.

I was overwhelmed with tears with the thought that Cooper had made it; it meant so much. Shortly after the phone call Cooper's surgeon came into the waiting room to tell me about his procedure.

"Cooper's was a very complicated and complex surgery. We had to reinstate life support on three different occasions. Cooper had a leak that we thought was coming from the patch but that wasn't what it was. He has a small mid-muscular defect (a hole in the muscle). It shouldn't be a problem and will heal on its own. We had to also use stainless steel wires to reattach his sternum."

After hearing the news I asked when I would be able to see Cooper. The doctor told me to give them fifteen minutes to get him settled and hooked up to the respirator and monitors.

When the doctor left, I sighed in relief that everything was okay. Mom told me that she sees a totally different person now that Cooper is okay and that now I didn't have to worry. Having my parents there by my side made me feel better, and the support they gave me through this whole thing meant more than words can describe. I was just glad I didn't have to go through this whole thing totally alone.

Fifteen minutes had passed and it was now time to see my son. I was scared because I had no idea what he would look like or the condition he would be in. Little did I know that the sight I was about to see would be the scariest and saddest sight in which a parent should ever have to see their child.

There was my son lying on a bed hooked to a respirator, chest tubes, pacemaker, and a monitor. I never once imagined I would ever see this. Cooper looked so helpless and fragile I just wanted to pick him up and hold him, but I knew I couldn't.

I stayed and visited for an hour, then went to the Ronald McDonald House for the night with my parents. So far, Cooper had been in the hospital for three weeks and it had been a very long three weeks.

A day after Cooper's surgery my parents had to head home. Before they did I spent some quality time with them alone to try to relax and enjoy myself a little. My parents took me for a ride out of the Portland area, down to the coast. We went out for lunch and even to Wal-Mart. We wanted to buy Cooper a get-well-soon balloon, but you were allowed to have only the aluminum balloons and the store didn't carry any. Instead, my mom and dad bought Cooper two really nice outfits. One was a precious moments coat and pant set, and the other was a white-and-blue sweater with a pair of tan-colored jeans with blue trim on the bottom of them. As we left Wal-Mart, I thanked my parents for everything they had done and for being there for both me and my son. I explained to them how much it meant to me and that I was very grateful. When we arrived back at the hospital I gave my parents a hug and kiss goodbye as they began to take their long journey back home.

Before I went into the hospital I went quickly to the Ronald McDonald House to drop off Cooper's clothes and to get a drink. The days passed by quickly and Cooper slowly began to decline in different areas. Four days after Cooper's surgery they tried to take him off the respirator but failed three different times before he finally got off. Then, spontaneously, Cooper had a 103 temperature and needed antibiotics.

I kept asking myself, What else will go wrong? I just wanted my son to be okay. He had been through too much already. I couldn't bear the thought of anything else going wrong. After five days of being hooked up to machines, I asked the nurse if

I could hold Cooper. I missed holding him in my arms and I wanted him to know that Mommy was there. The nurse set up a chair next to his bed and let me hold him.

It felt so comforting after a little less than a week of not being able to hold my son. When I held him in my arms, tears of joy began to flow. I kissed Cooper on the forehead and told him that Mamma was here. I rocked him gently in a rocking chair as I kept a close eye on his monitors to make sure I wouldn't set off his alarms.

Cooper was so sedated and light, it was like I was holding a lifeless animal in my arms. As I held Cooper close to my chest, all I could think about was how badly I wanted him to be able to get out of the ICU and back up to the Barbara Bush Wing.

Within days Cooper finally got to go back to his wing. I was extremely excited. Cooper was doing an excellent job and was being more lovable and sociable. He was starting to cry more and was beginning to be a very happy baby.

Things were really starting to look up and Cooper was being such a strong little guy. He showed me how to never give up and that by his fighting so much to stay here on Earth, I knew he was sent to me from above for a special reason.

Cooper is my miracle baby and has such a fighting instinct to stay alive. I knew that what the future would have in store for both of us would be a long, hard journey, but well worth it as long as we stayed by one another's side.

I was so excited that Cooper was going back to his wing that I went up there to tell his nurses that Cooper would soon be back and that it would be sometime that day. They were all excited and couldn't wait to see him again.

When we finally got back to the wing, I asked the doctor if they had any idea of how long Cooper would still be in the hospital. The doctor told me that if everything continued to go well and Cooper gained weight that in a week Cooper could be discharged.

Two days later I met up with Cooper's surgeon. He told me that Cooper was doing very well and that his incision was healing really well. Before I knew it, the appointed day for us to go home arrived. I was so excited I couldn't wait any longer. By 12:00 noon Cooper was discharged. Instead of taking a bus back home, Life Flight volunteered to fly us back home taking only two hours instead of a bus ride, which would have taken us over four hours plus a two-hour wait, only to have another four-to five-hour bus ride ahead of us.

Cooper's airplane experience was one he didn't care for too much. In between crying and sleeping I knew that soon we'd be arriving home. As for me, I didn't care too much for the ride either, but I knew I'd be home in a lot less time than if we were to have taken the bus.

When we finally landed in Caribou, Maine, I was so excited. My friend Kelley picked up Cooper and me from the airport. We went to her house and visited for a while. It felt good after being a month away from friends to finally be local and home.

As the days passed by, I had no idea of what the weeks or even months would turn out to be like for us. I was scared for a while to pick up Cooper because I thought I would hurt him.

Cooper's feedings began to slowly pick up, but as for his weight gaining, it began to become more of a struggle.

Before I knew it, Cooper's hectic schedule of activities began to take place. He had one to two appointments a week down state for follow-up visits. Then in December, at four months Cooper had a Child Developmental Clinic meeting, where a team of people would get together and assess Cooper to figure out what his needs would be. That day was a very long day that lasted at least four hours. Cooper had met with many different people who included the following:

1) A nursing assessment where he met with a nurse and me to discuss any allergies and his health. Cooper at the time of the meeting was a delightful baby and so happy. I informed the nurse about his cardiac situation and how he was on a spe-

cial formula called Enfamil 22 Calorie Formula to help with his weight gain.

This part of the assessment was hard because the nurse was telling me to try changing the size of Cooper's nipple because he wasn't taking very much formula. It didn't matter, because my son never really was a big eater and it didn't really bother me about what nipple to use because he had used so many different kinds anyway.

2) A medical evaluation was performed at this time where we went over topics like my background information, Cooper's hospital records, information from his pediatrician, copies of his chromosomal analysis, information from the Eastern Maine Medical Center as well as Cooper's surgical reports and information from his cardiologists.

During this part of our meeting, I was cool discussing everything that involved my son's special care he had received since birth, but when it came down to the point where I had to go into detail about what my childhood was like and how my parents were to my siblings, I felt it was too personal for them to know, but knew I had to cooperate with them.

3) A speech and language evaluation was performed on Cooper. They performed a test called a Receptive-Expressive Emergent Language Scale test, also known as REELS-2. Cooper's test results at this time for his receptive, expressive, as

well as overall emergent language skills, were consistent with a three-to four-month-old.

Cooper recognized facial expressions and would turn when I spoke. Cooper also would laugh and smile as well as initiate vocalization in an effort to get others to interact with him. Cooper would use two to three different sound syllables at a time. Whenever he was alone, Cooper would make noises and vocal sounds regardless of whether others were around or not.

Also at this time another test was performed called the Early Language Milestone Scale, also known as ELMS-2. This test placed Cooper's auditory receptive and auditory receptive language skills at a four-month age level.

4) A physical therapy evaluation was performed. In this evaluation Cooper was tested in five areas and they are as follows:

-<u>Musculoskeletal</u>: Cooper has a low level of muscle tone overall with hypermobility especially noted in the hip joints. On his back, Cooper tends to have lower extremities held in an externally rotated abducted position (frog leg) and arms also held externally rotated, abducted resting on the mat. When stimulated with a toy, he moves his arms and legs out of that position.

-<u>Gross Motor Skills</u>: The Peabody Developmental Motor Scale-2 (the PDMS-2) tests Cooper and measures his interrelated motor abilities that develop early in life. It is designed to assess the motor skills in children from birth to six years of age.

-<u>Reflexes</u>: The 8-item reflexes subtest measures aspects of a child's ability to automatically react to environmental events. Because reflexes typically become integrated by the time a child is 12 months old, this subtest is given only to children from birth through 11 months of age.

Cooper received a standard score of 8, which fell within the average range of 8–12. This put him at around a 1-month age level and at the 25% rank.

-<u>Stationary Skills</u>: This subtest measures the child's ability to control his or her body within its center of gravity and retain balance. It begins with simple activities such as head control in an infant, and progresses to higher-level activities of sitting and standing balance skills.

Cooper received a standard score of 6, which falls in the below average category and places him at a 1-month age equivalence. This represents a delay of 3 months in this area as well.

-<u>Locomotion</u>: This subtest measures the child's ability to move around in various forms. It also begins with infant activities, such as rolling and kicking legs, and increases in difficulty to higher level activities of walking, running, jumping, hopping, and skipping.

Cooper received a standard score of 7, which falls in the below average range and places him at a 1-month age equivalence. This represents a delay of 3 months.

5) An Occupational Therapy Evaluation was performed. This test as well was used with the PDMS-2 scale in six subtests.

-<u>Grasping</u>: This measures a child's ability to use his or her hands. It begins with the ability to hold an object with one hand and progresses to actions involving the controlled use of the fingers of both hands.

Cooper received a standard score of 7 in this subtest, which places him in the below average performance range. When placing a rattle in his hand, he was able to hold onto it between 15 and 29 seconds and was noted to move the rattle between 5 and 14 degrees. At this point, Cooper was not able to get the rattle when it was placed in front of him.

-<u>Visual Motor Integration</u>: This subtest measures a child's ability to use his or her visual perceptual skills to perform complex eye/hand coordination tasks, such as reaching and grasping for an object, building with blocks and copying designs.

Cooper received a standard score of 6 in this subject, which places him in the below average performance range when compared to other children his age. At this evaluation Cooper was not able to track a ball left to right or right to left, nor was he able to track a rattle beyond midline.

The Bayley Mental Scale was administered in order to assess overall cognitive/sensorimotor functioning. On the Bayley Mental Scale, Cooper achieved a Mental Developmental Index score of 83. Given the accuracy of the Bayley in assessing an infant's development, the evaluator was 90% confident that the range of scores from 78–92 reflects Cooper's true performance. This score falls at the 13th percentile and within the low average range of cognitive functioning. Cooper's overall performance on the Bayley was also approximately equivalent to the average performance of a 3-month-old child.

Cooper was able to follow objects that were presented in front of him in vertical as well as horizontal directions and even turned his head as he was following objects. He also was beginning to vocalize by cooing when spoken to by others.

Cooper let others know his needs of pleasure and displeasure and eagerness through his vocalizations. He is not yet, however, imitating sounds that others make to him. Good visual habituation responses were also observed in the evaluator's play with Cooper.

When the testing was over we had a final team meeting where we discussed that Cooper would need O/T (occupational therapy), P/T (physical therapy), D/T (developmental therapy), and S/T (speech therapy). We started off slowly with only D/T and O/T once a week, then as time progressed it increased. Before I knew it, I needed a pocket planner for all of Cooper's appointments.

Also at the clinic, I was told to sign up Cooper for disability and that he could not be turned down. The thought that he would be able to be set for life with guaranteed money each month made me feel a little more at ease. Also it was good because while Cooper resides with me, his monthly income would be able to help me out with his personal items, clothes and food. I was also informed that Cooper would qualify for respite services, even though the hours and pay were unspecified at that time. Knowing that there was a program out there to help give parents a break when they need it felt good and I knew that at times the program would come in handy.

Eventually things got to the point where Cooper was starting to have O/T once a week, D/T once a week, a visit with the public health nurse once a week, a checkup with the doctor once a week, and a team meeting with my case worker at least once every two weeks.

Now his schedule is O/T twice a week, P/T twice a week, S/T one to two times a month, and D/T once a week. He sees his public health nurse once every two weeks, his case worker once every two weeks, not counting doctors' appointments and specialty appointments like cardiology checkups, the eye doctor, hearing doctor and the gastro/intestinal specialist.

Cooper has changed my life in so many ways but all for the best. I look at how far he has come and am so impressed with it all. He overcame in the battle of life or death and has made it as far as to do so well that his cardiologist told me that instead of being seen once every one to three months, now he needs to be seen only every six months.

Both his doctor and I are so impressed on how strong his heart is. The most exciting news I was told was when he informed me that he feels Cooper will never need another surgery.

To this day, Cooper's therapies have helped him so much in so many ways. I am so impressed on how strong he has gotten. He has overcome so many challenges in so little time. After only five months of physical therapy, Cooper can now sit up with no support. He can also remain on his hands and knees with no support for about one to two minutes.

And that's not all. Cooper has begun to commando crawl and I know in my heart it won't be long before he will be crawling around. Cooper can now say the words Momma, Dada, and Baba. And he can completely roll over from side to side and from his back to his stomach.

Cooper can also clap his hands, attempts to stand up on his own, as well as pull himself up while he is against things. He screams due to recognizing he has a voice, he's eating finger foods and table foods, and finally, while lying down he is able to put himself in a sitting position. Cooper also loves to put his hands over his mouth and make noises, he loves to rock himself in his car seat, and yes, taking off his socks, as well as bath time, where he gets to splash his hands and kick his feet in the water.

However, Cooper still does have some problems even to this day, but not even half as many as what he has already been through. At Cooper's eye doctor appointment, he was found to be far-sighted and will need glasses in the spring. They will also have to look at what they can do to help correct his astigmatism (rattlingness) of the eyes.

Cooper also has a problem with constipation and I am currently working with the doctors to figure out what more we can do to help Cooper. It gets to the point where Cooper hurts so badly and gets so cramped that you hear nothing but bloody screams coming from the child. You can't help but want to cry and hold him while he hurts.

As for Cooper's feedings, they have gotten to the point where he loves to eat. He can eat foods with mixed textures and even loves his table foods. Cooper's weight has overcome the struggle as well, with him now weighing in at a remarkable sixteen pounds.

Cooper is so lovable and is such a happy baby. He loves being held and meeting new people. Cooper loves animals and is always laughing, talking, and smiling. I couldn't have asked for a better child. I know now that I was never once to blame for anything that happened to Cooper. He is a special child that God has given to me for a reason and he would never give me anything that he knew I would not be able to handle.

To this day, I enjoy my life with my son and really look forward to the future. Even though at this time Cooper is only about three to five months behind in learning, I know that he will do fine. As time goes on, I will learn so much more from both Cooper and his therapies as well as what Down Syndrome is. But for now, I finish this book with one final saying and I strongly recommend every parent to find the following book and CD.

The following sayings are bits and pieces from the CD. I hope it will hit home to you like it has for me and God bless you, your family, and especially your special angel.

From Bruce Carroll's book *Sometimes Miracles Hide*

"Sometimes miracles hide, God will wrap some blessings in disguise, you may have to wait this lifetime to see the reasons with your eyes, 'cause sometimes miracles hide. Though she was not like the other girls, they thought she was the best and through all the years of struggle, neither whispered one regret. See, to them it did not matter why some things in life take place, they just knew the joy they felt when they looked into her face."

978-0-595-37403-8
0-595-37403-4